EHLERS DANLOS SYNDROME

Unravelling the Mystery of Ehlers Danlos Syndrome

BY DR MILES JONES

INTRODUCTION

- *Definition of Ehlers Danlos Syndrome*
- *History and background of EDS*
- *Prevalence and incidence of EDS*

UNDERSTANDING EDS

- *Types of EDS and their symptoms*
- *Genetics and inheritance of EDS*
- *Diagnosis of EDS*
- *Misdiagnosis and comorbid conditions*

LIVING WITH EDS

- *Coping with chronic pain and fatigue*
- *Managing hypermobility and joint instability*
- *Lifestyle modifications and adaptations*
- *Psychological and social aspects of EDS*

MEDICAL MANAGEMENT OF EDS

- *Medications for pain, inflammation, and other symptoms*
- *Physical therapy and rehabilitation*
- *Orthotics and bracing*
- *Surgical options for joint stabilisation*

RESEARCH AND FUTURE DIRECTIONS

- *Current research on EDS*
- *Emerging therapies and treatments*
- *Advocacy and awareness efforts*

RESOURCES AND SUPPORT

- *Support groups and forums*
- *Tips for navigating the healthcare system*
- *Helpful tools and resources for daily living*

CONCLUSION

- *The impact of EDS on individuals and families*
- *Hope for the future*

INTRODUCTION

Definition of Ehlers Danlos Syndrome

Ehlers Danlos Syndrome (EDS) is a group of inherited genetic disorders that affect the body's connective tissues, which are responsible for providing support and structure to various organs and tissues. There are currently 13 recognized subtypes of EDS, each with its own specific set of symptoms and genetic mutations.

The most common symptoms of EDS include hypermobility of the joints, skin that is easily bruised and stretches easily, and a tendency toward chronic pain and fatigue. Other possible symptoms can include weak blood vessels and organs, scoliosis, flat feet, and dental problems.

EDS is caused by mutations in genes that are responsible for producing various types of collagen, which is a crucial component of connective tissue. The inheritance pattern of EDS varies depending on the subtype, but most forms are inherited in an autosomal dominant manner, meaning that a person only needs to inherit one copy of the mutated gene to develop the condition.

There is currently no cure for EDS, and treatment is focused on managing symptoms and preventing complications. This may include physical therapy, medication, and surgical interventions in severe cases.

History and background of EDS

Ehlers-Danlos Syndrome (EDS) is a group of genetic disorders that affect the connective tissues in the body. These disorders were first described by two physicians, Edvard Ehlers and Henri-Alexandre Danlos, in the early 1900s.

Ehlers was a Danish dermatologist who first identified a case of what he called "cutis laxa" in 1899. He observed a patient with loose and sagging skin, hypermobile joints, and fragile blood vessels. In 1901, he published a paper describing two more cases of the condition and coined the term "cutis laxa."

Danlos was a French dermatologist who observed similar symptoms in his patients and published his findings in 1908. He described a group of patients with skin that was stretchy and elastic, joints that were hypermobile, and a tendency towards easy bruising.

Over time, researchers began to realise that Ehlers and Danlos had identified two different forms of the same disorder. In 1956, the two types were officially classified as Ehlers-Danlos Syndrome, and additional types were identified as more research was conducted.

Currently, there are thirteen recognized subtypes of EDS, each with its own set of symptoms and genetic causes. The most common subtype is hypermobility-type EDS, which is characterised by joint hypermobility, skin that is soft and stretchy, and easy bruising. Other subtypes include classical EDS, vascular EDS, and kyphoscoliotic EDS, among others.

EDS is a rare disorder, and estimates suggest that it affects between 1 in 2,500 to 1 in 5,000 people worldwide.

Prevalence and incidence of EDS

Ehlers-Danlos Syndrome, is a group of genetic connective tissue disorders that affect the structure and function of various parts of the body, including the skin, joints, and blood vessels. There are currently 13 recognized subtypes of EDS, each with its own unique set of symptoms and diagnostic criteria.

The prevalence of EDS varies depending on the subtype. The most common subtype is the hypermobile type, which is estimated to affect 1 in 5,000 people worldwide. The classical type, which is characterised by skin hyperextensibility and joint hypermobility, is less common and has an estimatod prevalence of 1 in 20,000 to 1 in 40,000 people.

The incidence of EDS is difficult to determine because it is a genetic disorder that can be inherited in an autosomal dominant or recessive manner, or arise spontaneously due to a de novo mutation. However, studies have suggested that the incidence of EDS is likely higher than previously thought, with some estimates suggesting that up to 1 in 2,500 individuals may have some form of the condition.

It is important to note that EDS is a rare disorder, and many cases go undiagnosed or misdiagnosed due to its variable presentation and overlap with other conditions. If you suspect that you or a loved one may have EDS, it is important to speak with a healthcare professional who is familiar with the condition and can provide an accurate diagnosis and appropriate treatment.

UNDERSTANDING EDS

Types of EDS and their symptoms

EDS, or Ehlers-Danlos Syndrome, is a group of inherited connective tissue disorders that affect the body's ability to produce collagen, a protein that provides strength and elasticity to the skin, ligaments, and other tissues. There are 13 subtypes of EDS, each with its own unique set of symptoms and inheritance patterns. Here are brief descriptions of the most common subtypes and their symptoms:

Classical EDS: This type of EDS is characterised by hypermobility of the joints, skin that is easily bruised and stretches easily, and fragility of blood vessels and internal organs. Other symptoms include joint pain, scoliosis, flat feet, and poor wound healing.

Hypermobility EDS: This type of EDS is characterised by hypermobility of the joints and stretchy skin, but without the fragility of blood vessels seen in classical EDS. Other symptoms include chronic joint pain, fatigue, digestive issues, and dysautonomia (a malfunction of the autonomic nervous system).

Vascular EDS: This type of EDS is the most severe form and is characterised by thin, translucent skin that bruises easily, arterial and organ rupture, and a risk of life-threatening complications. Other symptoms include joint hypermobility, chronic joint pain, and hypermobility of blood vessels.

Kyphoscoliosis EDS: This type of EDS is characterised by severe curvature of the spine (kyphoscoliosis), joint hypermobility, and muscle weakness. Other symptoms include respiratory problems, vision problems, and fragile blood vessels.

Arthrochalasia EDS: This type of EDS is characterised by joint hypermobility, dislocations, and a risk of bone fractures. Other symptoms include scoliosis, muscle weakness, and stretchy skin.

Dermatosparaxis EDS: This type of EDS is characterised by extremely fragile skin that tears easily and is prone to scarring. Other symptoms include joint hypermobility, hernias, and short stature.

Brittle Cornea Syndrome: This type of EDS is characterised by thinning and rupture of the cornea, joint hypermobility, and stretchy skin. Other symptoms include nearsightedness and glaucoma.

It's important to note that some individuals may not fit neatly into one specific subtype and may exhibit a combination of symptoms from multiple subtypes. A geneticist or other healthcare professional with expertise in EDS can provide a proper diagnosis and treatment plan.

Genetics and inheritance of EDS

Ehlers-Danlos syndrome (EDS) is a group of inherited connective tissue disorders that affect the body's ability to produce or maintain strong, healthy collagen, which is a key component of many tissues in the body, including the skin, joints, and blood vessels.

EDS is typically inherited in an autosomal dominant pattern, which means that a person only needs to inherit one copy of the mutated gene from either parent in order to develop the condition. In some cases, however, EDS can be inherited in an autosomal recessive pattern, which means that a person must inherit two copies of the mutated gene (one from each parent) in order to develop the condition.

There are several different types of EDS, each of which is caused by mutations in different genes that affect the production or structure of collagen. For example, the most common type of EDS (known as hypermobile EDS) is caused by mutations in the

COL5A1 and COL5A2 genes, which are involved in the production of type V collagen.

In some cases, EDS can also occur sporadically, meaning that there is no family history of the condition. This can happen if a new mutation occurs spontaneously in a person's genes during their development.

Overall, the genetics of EDS are complex, and different types of EDS can be caused by mutations in different genes. Genetic testing may be helpful in diagnosing EDS and identifying the specific type of the condition. Genetic counselling can also be beneficial for individuals and families who are at risk of inheriting EDS or who have been diagnosed with the condition.

Diagnosis of EDS

Here are some steps that may be involved in the diagnosis of EDS:

1. Medical history: The doctor may ask questions about your symptoms, family history, and other medical conditions.

2. Physical exam: The doctor will examine your skin, joints, and other connective tissue. They may also test your flexibility and range of motion.

3. Genetic testing: A blood test can be done to identify genetic mutations that cause EDS.

4. Skin biopsy: A small sample of skin may be taken to examine the connective tissue under a microscope.

5. Imaging tests: X-rays, MRIs, or other imaging tests may be used to examine the joints, bones, and other tissues.

6. Cardiac testing: Depending on the type of EDS suspected, the doctor may perform cardiac tests to evaluate the function of the heart and blood vessels.

It's important to see a specialist who has experience with EDS for an accurate diagnosis.

Treatment options will vary depending on the type and severity of EDS.

Misdiagnosis and comorbid conditions

Misdiagnosis occurs when a medical condition is incorrectly identified or diagnosed. This can happen for various reasons, such as inadequate information, misinterpretation of test results, or the presence of comorbid conditions. Comorbid conditions refer to the presence of two or more medical conditions in the same person.

Comorbid conditions can complicate the diagnostic process because they can present symptoms that overlap with other conditions, leading to misdiagnosis.

Misdiagnosis can occur because many of the symptoms of EDS overlap with other conditions, such as chronic fatigue syndrome, fibromyalgia, and autoimmune disorders. Additionally, EDS can present with a wide range of symptoms and severity, making it challenging to diagnose.

Comorbid conditions, or conditions that occur alongside EDS, are also common. These can include:

1. Postural orthostatic tachycardia syndrome (POTS): This condition causes a rapid heart rate and dizziness upon standing. POTS is often seen in individuals with EDS due to autonomic dysfunction.

2. Mast cell activation syndrome (MCAS): MCAS is a condition where mast cells release too many chemical mediators, causing allergic-type symptoms. MCAS is more prevalent in individuals with EDS.

3. Gastrointestinal issues: EDS can cause digestive issues such as gastroparesis, irritable bowel syndrome, and inflammatory bowel disease.

4. Chronic pain: EDS is often associated with chronic pain, including joint pain, muscle pain, and headaches.

5. Anxiety and depression: Individuals with EDS may be more likely to experience anxiety and depression due to the impact of their condition on their daily life.

6. Sleep disorders: EDS can cause sleep disturbances, including insomnia and sleep apnea.

It's important for individuals with EDS to receive a comprehensive evaluation from a healthcare provider familiar with the condition. This can help ensure accurate diagnosis and management of both EDS and any comorbid conditions.

LIVING WITH EDS

Coping with chronic pain and fatigue

Coping with chronic pain and fatigue can be a significant challenge for individuals with Ehlers-Danlos syndrome (EDS). Here are some tips and strategies that may be helpful:

1. Develop a pain management plan: Work with your healthcare provider to develop a comprehensive pain management plan that includes medication, physical therapy, and alternative treatments like acupuncture or massage therapy.

2. Prioritise rest: Fatigue is a common symptom of EDS, so it is essential to prioritise rest. Pace yourself throughout the day and take breaks when you need them. If possible, try to establish a consistent sleep routine.

3. Engage in gentle exercise: Gentle exercise, such as yoga or swimming, can be helpful in managing pain and fatigue. Talk to your healthcare provider before starting any exercise program.

4. Manage stress: Stress can exacerbate pain and fatigue, so it is crucial to find ways to manage stress. Consider mindfulness meditation, deep breathing exercises, or therapy to help manage stress.

5. Seek support: Living with chronic pain and fatigue can be isolating, so it is essential to seek support. Consider joining a support group or reaching out to friends and family for support.

6. Modify your environment: Modifying your environment can help you conserve energy and reduce pain. Consider using ergonomic tools, such as a standing desk or an ergonomic keyboard, to reduce strain on your body.

7. Practise good self-care: Good self-care, such as eating a healthy diet, staying hydrated, and avoiding smoking, can help manage pain and fatigue.

Remember, managing chronic pain and fatigue is a process, and it may take time to find what works best for you. Be patient with yourself and work with your healthcare provider to develop a plan that meets your needs.

Managing hypermobility and joint instability

Ehlers-Danlos Syndrome (EDS) is a genetic disorder that affects the connective tissue in the body, leading to joint hypermobility, joint instability, and other symptoms. Here are some tips for managing hypermobility and joint instability in EDS:

1. Physical therapy: Working with a physical therapist can help strengthen muscles around the joints and improve joint stability. Your physical therapist may also recommend specific exercises to improve joint range of motion and prevent injury.

2. Bracing: Joint braces or compression garments can provide additional support to unstable joints, especially during physical activity.

3. Avoid overextending joints: It is important to avoid activities or positions that may cause excessive strain on the joints. Activities that involve repetitive impact or twisting motions, such as running or tennis, should be avoided or modified.

4. Maintain a healthy weight: Excess weight can put additional stress on the joints, so

maintaining a healthy weight can help reduce joint pain and improve joint stability.

5. Joint protection: Simple techniques like avoiding prolonged standing or sitting, taking frequent breaks during physical activity, and using assistive devices (e.g., crutches, canes) can help reduce the stress on joints.

6. Pain management: Over-the-counter pain relievers like acetaminophen or nonsteroidal anti-inflammatory drugs (NSAIDs) can help manage joint pain. Your doctor may also prescribe stronger pain medication or recommend other pain management strategies.

7. Hydration and nutrition: Proper hydration and nutrition are important for maintaining healthy connective tissue. Drinking plenty of water and consuming a balanced diet rich in vitamins and minerals can help support joint health.

8. Stress management: Stress can exacerbate joint pain and other symptoms of EDS. Strategies such as mindfulness meditation, deep breathing, or talking to a mental health professional can help manage stress and improve overall well-being.

Lifestyle modifications and adaptations

Ehlers-Danlos Syndrome (EDS) is a rare genetic disorder that affects the body's connective tissue, which can lead to joint hypermobility, skin that stretches easily, and other symptoms. While there is no cure for EDS, lifestyle modifications and adaptations can help manage symptoms and improve quality of life. Here are some lifestyle modifications and adaptations that can be beneficial for individuals with EDS:

Exercise: Regular exercise can help strengthen muscles and improve joint stability. Low-impact exercises such as swimming, walking, and yoga can be beneficial.

Diet: Eating a balanced and nutritious diet can help maintain a healthy weight and support overall health. Avoiding inflammatory foods such as processed foods and sugar can also be beneficial.

Sleep: Getting enough restful sleep is important for individuals with EDS. Developing good sleep habits such as maintaining a regular sleep schedule, avoiding caffeine and electronics before bedtime, and creating a comfortable sleep environment can help improve sleep quality.

Joint protection: Individuals with EDS are more prone to joint dislocations and injuries. Wearing braces or splints, using assistive devices such as canes or crutches, and avoiding high-impact activities can help protect joints.

Stress management: Stress can worsen EDS symptoms, so it's important to develop healthy stress management techniques such as meditation, deep breathing, or yoga.

Occupational therapy: Occupational therapy can help individuals with EDS learn how to perform daily tasks in a way that minimises joint strain and injury.

Pain management: Chronic pain is a common symptom of EDS. Pain management techniques such as physical therapy, medication, and alternative therapies like acupuncture or massage can help manage pain.

Mental health support: Coping with a chronic illness can be challenging. Seeking support from a mental health professional or joining a support group can help individuals with EDS manage their emotions and improve their quality of life.

Psychological and social aspects of EDS

The psychological and social aspects of EDS can have a significant impact on individuals living with this condition.

Here are some of the psychological and social aspects of EDS:

Chronic pain: Many individuals with EDS experience chronic pain, which can have a profound effect on their psychological well-being. Chronic pain can cause anxiety, depression, and other mood disorders.

Anxiety and depression: The physical limitations and unpredictability of symptoms can cause anxiety and depression in individuals with EDS. They may worry about their future, their ability to work, and their quality of life.

Social isolation: Some individuals with EDS may feel socially isolated due to their physical limitations. They may have difficulty participating in activities with friends and family, which can lead to feelings of loneliness and isolation.

Stigma and misconceptions: There are many misconceptions about EDS, which can lead to stigma and discrimination. Some people may assume that individuals with EDS are lazy or exaggerating their symptoms.

Coping mechanisms: Individuals with EDS may develop coping mechanisms to deal with their symptoms. These may include avoiding certain activities or relying on pain medication. These coping mechanisms can have both positive and negative effects on their psychological well-being.

Support systems: Support from friends, family, and healthcare providers is crucial for individuals with EDS. Support can help individuals feel less isolated and provide them with resources and information to manage their symptoms.

Overall, the psychological and social aspects of EDS can be challenging for individuals living with this condition. It is important for individuals with EDS to seek support from healthcare providers, support groups, and loved ones to help them manage their symptoms and improve their quality of life.

MEDICAL MANAGEMENT OF EDS

Medications for pain, inflammation, and other symptoms

Ehlers-Danlos Syndrome (EDS) is a genetic disorder that affects the connective tissue in the body. It can cause a wide range of symptoms, including chronic pain and inflammation. While there is no cure for EDS, medications can be used to manage these symptoms and improve quality of life.

Here are some medications that may be used for pain, inflammation, and other symptoms in EDS:

Nonsteroidal anti-inflammatory drugs (NSAIDs): NSAIDs like ibuprofen and naproxen can help reduce pain and inflammation in EDS. However, they should be used with caution, as they can cause stomach irritation and increase the risk of bleeding.

Acetaminophen: Acetaminophen is a pain reliever that does not have anti-inflammatory properties. It is generally considered safe for people with EDS, but it should not be used in high doses or for long periods of time.

Opioids: Opioids like morphine and oxycodone are strong pain relievers that can be used for severe pain in EDS. However, they are highly addictive and can cause serious side effects, so they should only be used under the guidance of a healthcare provider.

Antidepressants: Tricyclic antidepressants like amitriptyline and nortriptyline can be used to treat chronic pain in EDS. They work by changing the way the brain perceives pain.

Anticonvulsants: Anticonvulsants like gabapentin and pregabalin can also be used to treat chronic pain in EDS. They work by blocking the transmission of pain signals in the brain.

Muscle relaxants: Muscle relaxants like baclofen and tizanidine can help relieve muscle spasms and tightness in EDS.

It's important to note that medications should only be used under the guidance of a healthcare provider, and that they may not be effective for everyone with EDS. Other treatments, such as physical therapy and lifestyle changes, may also be recommended to manage symptoms.

Physical therapy and rehabilitation

Ehlers-Danlos Syndrome (EDS) is a rare genetic disorder that affects the connective tissues in the body. It is characterised by hypermobility, joint instability, and a range of other symptoms that can severely impact a person's quality of life. Physical therapy and rehabilitation can play a crucial role in managing the symptoms of EDS and improving the functional abilities of individuals living with this condition.

Physical therapy is a branch of healthcare that focuses on helping people recover from injury or manage chronic conditions through exercise, manual therapy, and other non-invasive treatments. In the case of EDS, physical therapy can help individuals improve their muscle strength, stability, and range of motion, as well as manage pain and prevent further joint damage.

One of the most important aspects of physical therapy for EDS is strengthening the muscles around the joints. When the ligaments and tendons that support the joints are weak, it can lead to joint instability and pain. Physical therapists can design exercises that target the specific muscle groups needed to stabilise the joints, such as the core, hip, and shoulder muscles. These exercises can be done at home or in a supervised setting, depending on the individual's needs.

Another key area of focus for physical therapy in EDS is improving posture and body mechanics. Poor posture can put unnecessary strain on the joints and exacerbate pain and other symptoms. Physical therapists can teach individuals how to sit, stand, and move in ways that minimise stress on the joints and improve overall alignment. They may also recommend assistive devices, such as braces or orthotics, to help support the joints and improve mobility.

In addition to exercise and manual therapy, physical therapists may use other modalities to manage pain and inflammation in individuals with EDS. These may include ice or heat therapy, electrical stimulation, or ultrasound. They may also provide education on lifestyle modifications, such as avoiding certain activities or using adaptive equipment, to prevent further joint damage.

Rehabilitation is another important component of managing EDS. Rehabilitation refers to a range of services that help individuals regain functional abilities and independence after injury or illness. In the case of EDS, rehabilitation may be necessary after joint surgeries or other interventions.

Rehabilitation for EDS can include physical therapy, occupational therapy, and speech therapy, depending on the individual's needs. Occupational therapy focuses on helping individuals perform activities of daily living, such as bathing, dressing, and cooking, while minimising stress on the joints. Speech therapy can help individuals with EDS who have swallowing difficulties or other speech-related issues.

Rehabilitation can also include psychological support, such as counselling or cognitive-behavioural therapy. Living with a chronic condition like EDS can be challenging, and many individuals may experience anxiety, depression, or other mental health concerns. Rehabilitation services can help individuals develop coping strategies and improve their overall well-being.

In conclusion, physical therapy and rehabilitation are essential components of managing Ehlers-Danlos Syndrome. These services can help individuals improve their muscle strength, joint stability, and range of motion, as well as manage pain and prevent further joint damage. With the right support, individuals with EDS can maintain their functional abilities and independence, improving their quality of life and overall health.

Orthotics and bracing

Orthotics and bracing are commonly used in the management of Ehlers-Danlos Syndrome (EDS), a group of genetic disorders that affect the connective tissues in the body. EDS can cause a range of symptoms, including joint hypermobility, chronic pain, and skin fragility. Orthotics and bracing are designed to support and stabilise affected joints, reduce pain, and improve function in individuals with EDS.

Orthotics are medical devices that are worn on the body to correct or alleviate musculoskeletal problems. In EDS, orthotics are commonly used to support unstable joints, particularly those in the ankles, knees, hips, and spine. Orthotics can also be used to correct joint deformities, such as scoliosis, or to improve balance and gait. There are many different types of orthotics, including shoe inserts, ankle braces, knee braces, spinal braces, and wrist splints.

Shoe inserts are one of the most common types of orthotics used in EDS. They are designed to improve foot alignment and reduce the risk of foot and ankle injuries. Inserts can be custom-made to fit the individual's foot and provide specific support in areas of weakness or instability. Ankle braces are another common type of orthotic used in EDS. They are designed to support the ankle joint and prevent excessive movement that can lead to sprains or other injuries. Ankle braces can be made from a variety of materials, including neoprene, plastic, and metal.

Knee braces are another common type of orthotic used in EDS. They are designed to support the knee joint and reduce pain and instability. Knee braces can be designed to stabilise the joint in a specific direction, such as medial or lateral, or to provide overall support to the joint. Spinal braces are used in individuals with EDS who have scoliosis or other spinal deformities. These braces are designed to correct the curvature of the spine and prevent further progression of the deformity. Wrist splints are another common type of orthotic used in EDS. They are designed to support the wrist joint and reduce pain and instability.

Bracing is a term used to describe the use of external supports to stabilise joints and prevent excessive movement. Bracing is commonly used in individuals with EDS who have joint hypermobility or instability. Braces can be made from a variety of materials, including neoprene, plastic, and metal. They can be designed to stabilise a specific joint or to provide overall support to the body. Braces are often used in combination with other treatments, such as physical therapy and medication, to manage symptoms of EDS.

One of the benefits of orthotics and bracing in EDS is their ability to improve joint stability and reduce pain. Orthotics and braces can also improve overall function and mobility, allowing individuals with EDS to perform daily activities with less difficulty and discomfort. However, orthotics and bracing are not without risks. They can cause skin irritation, pressure sores, and discomfort if they do not fit properly or are not used correctly. In addition, some individuals with EDS may not be able

Surgical options for joint stabilisation

Ehlers-Danlos Syndrome (EDS) is a group of genetic disorders that affect the body's connective tissues, leading to joint hypermobility, skin laxity, and other symptoms. Joint instability is a common feature of EDS, and can lead to pain, dislocations, and functional impairment. While non-surgical options such as physical therapy and bracing can be effective for some patients, in some cases surgical intervention may be necessary to stabilise joints and improve function. There are several surgical options for joint stabilisation in EDS, which I will discuss in more detail below.

Arthroscopic stabilisation is a minimally invasive surgical technique that can be used to stabilise certain joints in patients with EDS. This procedure involves making small incisions and using a camera and specialised instruments to repair damaged ligaments and other soft tissues that support the joint. Arthroscopic stabilisation is often used to treat shoulder instability, which is common in EDS patients, but can also be used for other joints such as the knee and ankle. While arthroscopic stabilisation is less invasive than open surgery, it is not always suitable for all patients, and may not provide long-lasting stability in some cases.

Open surgical stabilisation is another option for joint stabilisation in EDS patients. This involves making larger incisions and directly repairing or reconstructing damaged ligaments and other soft tissues. Open surgical stabilisation may be necessary for more severe cases of joint instability or for joints that are not amenable to arthroscopic stabilisation. This procedure may involve using grafts or other materials to reinforce the joint, and may require a longer recovery period than arthroscopic surgery.

Joint fusion is a more radical surgical option for joint stabilisation in EDS patients. This procedure involves permanently joining two or more bones together to create a stable joint. Joint fusion is typically reserved for cases of severe joint degeneration or instability that cannot be treated by other means. While joint fusion can provide long-lasting stability, it does sacrifice joint mobility, and may increase stress on adjacent joints, leading to further problems down the line.

Joint replacement is another option for joint stabilisation in EDS patients, particularly in cases of severe joint degeneration. This procedure involves replacing the damaged joint with an artificial joint made of metal, plastic, or ceramic components. Joint replacement can provide significant pain relief and improved function in patients with severe joint degeneration, but it is not always appropriate for EDS patients due to their increased risk of joint dislocations and other complications.

In addition to these surgical options, it is important for EDS patients to receive comprehensive pre- and post-operative care to minimise the risk of complications and optimise outcomes. This may include physical therapy, pain management, and ongoing monitoring of joint stability and function.

In summary, there are several surgical options available for joint stabilisation in EDS patients, ranging from minimally invasive arthroscopic stabilisation to more radical procedures such as joint fusion or replacement. The choice of procedure will depend on the severity of the joint instability, the specific joint involved, and the patient's individual needs and goals. It is important for EDS patients to work closely with a team of healthcare professionals to develop a personalised treatment plan that takes into account their unique needs and circumstances.

RESEARCH AND FUTURE DIRECTIONS

Current research on EDS

Current research on EDS focuses on several areas, including:

Genetics: Scientists are exploring the genetic causes of EDS and the mutations that lead to collagen production problems. Recent studies have identified new genes and mutations associated with EDS, which may lead to better diagnosis and treatment options.

Diagnosis and classification: Researchers are working to improve the diagnosis and classification of EDS, which can be challenging due to the wide range of symptoms and types of the disorder. Advances in imaging and genetic testing may help to improve accuracy and consistency in diagnosing EDS.

Treatment: There is currently no cure for EDS, and treatment primarily focuses on managing symptoms. Researchers are exploring new treatments, such as gene therapy and regenerative medicine, that may help to address the underlying causes of EDS and improve outcomes for patients.

Comorbidities: EDS is often associated with other conditions, such as dysautonomia, gastrointestinal disorders, and chronic pain. Researchers are investigating the links between EDS and these comorbidities to better understand how they are related and how they can be treated.

Overall, research on EDS is ongoing and multifaceted, with a focus on understanding the underlying causes of the disorder and developing new and more effective treatment options.

Emerging therapies and treatments

Ehlers-Danlos Syndrome (EDS) is a rare genetic disorder that affects the body's connective tissue. Connective tissue provides support to various body structures, including skin, bones, blood vessels, and internal organs. EDS can cause a wide range of symptoms, including joint hypermobility, skin hyperextensibility, chronic pain, and fatigue. Although there is no cure for EDS, there are various emerging therapies and treatments that can help manage the symptoms and improve quality of life for those living with the condition.

One emerging therapy for EDS is regenerative medicine. Regenerative medicine involves using stem cells or other types of cells to repair damaged tissues or organs. Some researchers are investigating the use of stem cells to repair damaged connective tissue in EDS patients. For example, a recent study found that stem cell therapy improved the biomechanical properties of skin in a mouse model of EDS. However, more research is needed to determine the safety and efficacy of stem cell therapy for EDS in humans.

Another emerging therapy for EDS is gene therapy. Gene therapy involves introducing healthy genes into the body to replace or repair damaged or missing genes. Researchers are investigating the use of gene therapy to treat various genetic disorders, including EDS. For example, a recent study found that gene therapy improved the collagen structure and skin mechanics in a mouse model of EDS. However, more research is needed to determine the safety and efficacy of gene therapy for EDS in humans.

Physical therapy and exercise are also important components of EDS management. Physical therapy can help improve joint stability and reduce pain in EDS patients. Some researchers are investigating the use of exercise therapy to improve muscle function and reduce joint hypermobility in EDS patients. For example, a recent study found that a specific exercise program improved muscle strength and balance in EDS patients.

Another emerging therapy for EDS is the use of medical devices, such as braces and compression garments. These devices can help support the joints and improve overall function in EDS patients. For example, a recent study found that a custom knee brace improves knee stability and reduces pain in EDS patients with knee instability.

Finally, there are various medications that can be used to manage specific symptoms of EDS. For example, nonsteroidal anti-inflammatory drugs (NSAIDs) can help reduce pain and inflammation in EDS patients. Some researchers are investigating the use of drugs that target specific biochemical pathways involved in EDS, such as the lysyl oxidase-like 1 (LOXL1) pathway. For example, a recent study found that an inhibitor of the LOXL1 pathway improved the biomechanical properties of skin in a mouse model of EDS.

In conclusion, while there is no cure for Ehlers-Danlos Syndrome, there are various emerging therapies and treatments that can help manage the symptoms and improve quality of life for those living with the condition. These include regenerative medicine, gene therapy, physical therapy and exercise, medical devices, and medications. However, more research is needed to determine the safety and efficacy of these treatments for EDS in humans.

Advocacy and awareness efforts

Ehlers-Danlos Syndrome (EDS) is a group of genetic disorders that affects the connective tissues in the body. EDS is a complex condition, and it can be difficult to diagnose, leading to misdiagnosis and delays in treatment. Advocacy and awareness efforts are critical in increasing understanding of EDS and improving diagnosis and treatment for those affected by the condition.

Advocacy efforts on EDS include a range of activities aimed at raising awareness, educating the public, and influencing policy. These efforts are typically led by patient advocacy groups, non-profit organisations, and individuals affected by EDS. Some common advocacy activities include:

Awareness campaigns: EDS awareness campaigns are designed to educate the public about the condition, its symptoms, and the challenges faced by those affected by the condition. These campaigns often involve social media outreach, public events, and community outreach.

Patient support groups: Patient support groups provide a platform for people with EDS to connect with others who are going through similar experiences. These groups offer emotional support, practical advice, and information about EDS.

Research funding: Advocacy organisations work to raise funds for EDS research, which can help to improve diagnosis and treatment for those affected by the condition. This funding can support research studies, clinical trials, and other projects aimed at improving understanding of EDS.

Legislative advocacy: Advocacy groups work to influence policy and legislative initiatives that affect people with EDS. These efforts may include lobbying for increased funding for research or advocating for changes in insurance coverage for EDS-related treatments.

Awareness efforts on EDS can also help to improve understanding of the condition among healthcare professionals, leading to earlier diagnosis and more effective treatment. In addition to advocacy efforts, there are a number of other strategies that can be used to increase awareness of EDS, including:

Social media outreach: Social media platforms provide a powerful tool for raising awareness of EDS. Advocacy organisations and individuals can use social media to share information about EDS, connect with others affected by the condition, and promote advocacy efforts.

Public events: Public events, such as conferences, seminars, and workshops, provide an opportunity to educate healthcare professionals, researchers, and the general public about EDS.

Educational resources: Educational resources, such as brochures, videos, and websites, can be used to provide information about EDS to healthcare professionals, patients, and the general public.

Patient testimonials: Patient testimonials can be a powerful tool for raising awareness of EDS. Sharing stories of individuals who have been affected by the condition can help to humanise the condition and promote empathy and understanding.

Advocacy and awareness efforts on EDS are critical in improving the lives of those affected by the condition. By increasing understanding of EDS and improving diagnosis and treatment, advocacy and awareness efforts can help to improve the quality of life for individuals with EDS and their families. If you or someone you know is affected by EDS, getting involved with advocacy and awareness efforts can be a powerful way to make a difference.

RESOURCES AND SUPPORT

Support groups and forums

Ehlers-Danlos Syndrome (EDS) is a rare genetic disorder that affects connective tissue, causing symptoms such as hypermobility, joint pain, skin fragility, and fatigue, among others. Living with EDS can be challenging, both physically and emotionally. This is where support groups and forums can play a vital role in the lives of those affected by EDS.

Support groups and forums provide a safe and welcoming space for individuals with EDS to connect with others who understand their condition and its impact on their lives. Through these groups, people can share their experiences, ask for advice, and receive emotional support from others who are going through similar struggles. Support groups and forums can be in-person, online, or a combination of both, depending on the preferences and needs of the participants.

One of the most significant benefits of support groups and forums for people with EDS is the sense of community they provide. EDS can be a lonely and isolating condition, especially when friends and family members don't fully understand what it's like to live with it. Support groups and forums offer a sense of belonging and connection to others who share similar experiences, providing a space where people can feel heard, understood, and validated.

Another benefit of support groups and forums is the wealth of knowledge and information they offer. Participants can learn from each other's experiences and share tips and strategies for managing symptoms and improving quality of life. This can include advice on everything from adaptive equipment and mobility aids to coping techniques for chronic pain and fatigue.

Support groups and forums can also be an excellent source of emotional support for people with EDS. Living with a chronic condition can take a toll on mental health, and having a supportive community can help alleviate feelings of anxiety, depression, and isolation. Support groups and forums can provide a safe and non-judgmental space for people to express their feelings, share their struggles, and receive encouragement from others who understand what they're going through.

In addition to providing emotional support and practical advice, support groups and forums can also be a powerful advocacy tool. By connecting with others who have similar experiences, participants can come together to raise awareness about EDS, advocate for better research and treatment options, and push for more accessible and inclusive healthcare policies.

Overall, support groups and forums can be an invaluable resource for individuals with EDS and their loved ones. By providing a sense of community, knowledge, and emotional support, these groups can help people with EDS feel less alone, better manage their symptoms, and advocate for themselves and their community. Whether online or in-person, support groups and forums are a powerful way to connect with others, learn from each other's experiences, and make a positive impact on the lives of those affected by EDS.

Tips for navigating the healthcare system

Ehlers-Danlos syndrome (EDS) is a rare genetic condition that affects the connective tissues in the body. It can cause a range of symptoms, from joint hypermobility and chronic pain to digestive issues and cardiovascular problems. Navigating the healthcare system with EDS can be challenging, but with the right strategies and resources, it can be manageable. Here are some tips for navigating the healthcare system with EDS:

1. Find a knowledgeable healthcare provider: One of the most important steps in managing EDS is finding a healthcare

provider who is knowledgeable about the condition. This may require some research, as EDS is a rare condition and not all healthcare providers are familiar with it. Look for a provider who specialises in EDS or has experience working with patients with the condition. They will be better equipped to provide you with the appropriate care and treatment options.

2. Build a healthcare team: EDS can affect multiple parts of the body, so it's important to have a healthcare team that includes specialists in different areas. This may include a rheumatologist, orthopedist, cardiologist, gastroenterologist, and pain management specialist, among others. Having a team of healthcare providers who are familiar with your condition can help ensure that all of your symptoms and needs are addressed.

3. Keep a medical history and symptom log: EDS can cause a wide range of symptoms, and it's important to keep track of them so that you can communicate effectively with your healthcare providers. Keep a log of your symptoms, when they occur, and how long they last. This can help your healthcare team identify patterns and develop a treatment plan that addresses your specific needs.

4. Advocate for yourself: Healthcare providers may not always be familiar with EDS, so it's important to advocate for yourself and your needs. Be prepared to educate your providers about the condition and how it affects you. Bring information about EDS to your appointments, and be proactive in communicating your symptoms and concerns.

5. Be prepared for appointments: Before your appointments, make a list of questions and concerns you want to discuss with your healthcare provider. Bring any medical records, test results, and other relevant information with you to the appointment. This can help ensure that your provider has all of the information they need to make informed decisions about your care.

6. Stay organised: Managing EDS can involve multiple appointments, medications, and treatments. Stay organised by keeping a calendar of appointments, a list of medications and dosages, and a record of treatments you've received. This can help you stay on top of your care and avoid missing appointments or doses of medication.

7. Connect with support groups: Living with EDS can be challenging, and it can be helpful to connect with others who are going through similar experiences. Look for support groups in your area or online. These groups can provide valuable information, emotional support, and a sense of community.

8. Take care of yourself: Managing EDS can be stressful, so it's important to take care of yourself. Practice self-care activities that help you relax and manage stress, such as meditation, yoga, or massage. Get regular exercise, eat a healthy diet, and get plenty of sleep. These habits can help you feel better and better manage your symptoms.

In conclusion, navigating the healthcare system with EDS can be challenging, but with the right strategies and resources, it can be manageable. Finding knowledgeable healthcare providers, building a healthcare team, keeping a medical history and symptom log, advocating for yourself, being prepared for appointments, staying organised, connecting with support groups, and taking care of yourself are all important strategies for managing EDS. By following these tips, you can better manage your condition and live a healthier, more fulfilling life.

Helpful tools and resources for daily living

Ehlers-Danlos Syndrome (EDS) is a genetic disorder that affects the body's connective tissue, causing it to become weak and fragile. This can lead to a wide range of symptoms, including joint hypermobility, chronic pain, easy bruising, and fatigue. Living with EDS can be challenging, but there are many helpful tools and resources available to make daily life more manageable.

1. Mobility aids: Many people with EDS experience joint hypermobility, which can lead to chronic pain and difficulty with movement. Mobility aids such as braces, canes, walkers, and wheelchairs can help support joints and improve mobility, making daily activities easier and less painful.

2. Adaptive equipment: Adaptive equipment such as shower chairs, raised toilet seats, and grab bars can make everyday tasks safer and more accessible for people with EDS. These tools can help prevent falls and reduce the risk of injury.

3. Pain management tools: Chronic pain is a common symptom of EDS. Pain management tools such as heating pads, ice packs, and TENS units can help reduce pain and improve quality of life.

4. Medication: In some cases, medication may be necessary to manage EDS symptoms. Your doctor can prescribe pain medication, anti-inflammatory medication, and other medications as needed.

5. Physical therapy: Physical therapy can help strengthen muscles, improve joint stability, and reduce pain in people with EDS. A physical therapist can work with you to develop a customised exercise plan that meets your specific needs.

6. Occupational therapy: Occupational therapy can help people with EDS learn strategies to manage daily tasks and improve their quality of life. An occupational therapist can help you develop strategies for managing pain, conserving energy, and adapting your environment to meet your needs.

7. Support groups: Support groups can provide a valuable source of emotional support and practical advice for people with EDS. Online and in-person support groups are available, allowing you to connect with others who understand what you're going through.

8. Counselling: Living with a chronic condition like EDS can be challenging, and

counselling can help you manage the emotional impact of your condition. A therapist can help you develop coping strategies, improve your self-esteem, and manage stress and anxiety.

9. Online resources: There are many online resources available for people with EDS, including websites, forums, and social media groups. These resources can provide valuable information, support, and advice.

10. Medical alert jewellery: Medical alert jewellery can be especially important for people with EDS, as the condition can affect multiple organ systems. Wearing a medical alert bracelet or necklace can alert emergency responders to your condition and any special needs you may have.

In conclusion, living with EDS can be challenging, but there are many tools and resources available to make daily life more manageable. Mobility aids, adaptive equipment, pain management tools, medication, physical therapy, occupational therapy, support groups, counselling, online resources, and medical alert jewellery can all play a valuable role in helping people with EDS live full and satisfying lives. It's important to work closely with your healthcare team to develop a comprehensive treatment plan that addresses all aspects of your condition.

CONCLUSION

The impact of EDS on individuals and families

Ehlers-Danlos Syndrome (EDS) is a group of rare genetic disorders that affect the connective tissues in the body, causing a wide range of symptoms and complications. The impact of EDS on individuals and families can be significant and multifaceted, affecting not only physical health but also emotional well-being, social relationships, and financial stability.

Physical Impact
EDS affects the connective tissues that support and connect various structures in the body, such as the skin, joints, and blood vessels. This can lead to a wide range of physical symptoms and complications, including joint hypermobility, chronic pain, fatigue, easy bruising and scarring, gastrointestinal problems, heart problems, and more. These symptoms can be severe and debilitating, affecting the ability of individuals to carry out daily activities, work, and participate in social and recreational activities.

Emotional Impact
Living with EDS can be emotionally challenging, as individuals may struggle with chronic pain, fatigue, and other physical symptoms, which can lead to depression, anxiety, and other mental health

conditions. Additionally, the uncertainty of the condition, the lack of awareness and understanding by others, and the difficulties accessing appropriate care can all contribute to feelings of isolation, frustration, and hopelessness.

Social Impact

The physical limitations imposed by EDS can also affect individuals' social lives and relationships. Many people with EDS report feeling isolated, as they are unable to participate in social activities or hobbies they once enjoyed. Additionally, the unpredictable nature of the condition can make it difficult for individuals to commit to plans or make long-term arrangements, leading to social anxiety and strained relationships.

Financial Impact

The financial impact of EDS can be significant, as individuals may require frequent medical care, specialised equipment, and accommodations to manage their symptoms and maintain their independence. Many people with EDS also struggle to work full-time or maintain employment due to their physical limitations, which can lead to financial instability and additional stress.

Impact on Family Members

The impact of EDS is not limited to the individual affected by the condition but also extends to their family members. Family members may take on additional responsibilities and caregiving duties, which can be physically and emotionally demanding. They may also experience feelings of helplessness and frustration as they try to support their loved one but struggle to find adequate resources and support.

Additionally, EDS is a genetic condition, which means that family members may also be at risk of developing the condition themselves. This can lead to additional anxiety and worry, as well as the need for increased monitoring and medical care.

Management and Support
While living with EDS can be challenging, there are ways to manage symptoms and improve quality of life. This may include a combination of medical treatments, such as physical therapy, pain management, and surgery, as well as lifestyle changes, such as exercise, nutrition, and stress management. Support groups and online communities can also provide valuable emotional support and a sense of community for individuals and their families.

In conclusion, the impact of EDS on individuals and families can be significant and multifaceted, affecting physical health, emotional well-being, social relationships, and financial stability. It is important for individuals with EDS and their families to have access to appropriate medical care and support to manage symptoms, improve quality of life, and cope with the challenges of living with this condition.

Hope for the future

Ehlers-Danlos Syndrome (EDS) is a genetic disorder that affects connective tissues in the body, including joints, skin, and blood vessels. It is a chronic condition that can cause a range of symptoms, including joint pain, skin hypermobility, and organ dysfunction. While there is currently no cure for EDS, there is hope for the future in terms of both treatment and research.

One of the reasons for hope in the treatment of EDS is the development of new therapies. While traditional treatments for EDS have focused on managing symptoms, such as pain medication and physical therapy, researchers are exploring new approaches that could target the underlying causes of the disorder. For example, gene therapy is a promising area of research that could potentially correct the genetic mutations that cause EDS. Another potential therapy is the use of stem cells to regenerate damaged connective tissues in the body. While these treatments are still in the early stages of development, they offer hope for future breakthroughs in the treatment of EDS.

In addition to new therapies, there is also hope for improved diagnosis and management of EDS. One of the challenges with EDS is that it can be difficult to diagnose, as symptoms can vary widely from person to person and can overlap with other conditions. However, advances in genetic testing and imaging technology are making it easier to identify the specific genetic mutations that cause EDS and to detect changes in connective tissues in the body. This could lead to earlier diagnosis and more targeted treatment.

There is also hope for improved management of EDS symptoms. While there is no cure for EDS, there are a number of lifestyle changes and therapies that can help manage symptoms and improve quality of life. For example, physical therapy and exercise can help strengthen joints and improve mobility, while medications such as nonsteroidal anti-inflammatory drugs (NSAIDs) can help manage pain and inflammation. Additionally, there are a range of assistive devices and adaptive technologies that can help individuals with EDS perform everyday tasks more easily.

Finally, there is hope for continued research into the underlying causes of EDS. While the genetic mutations that cause EDS are known, there is still much to learn about how these mutations affect connective tissues in the body. Researchers are exploring a range of questions, such as why some individuals with EDS experience more severe symptoms than others, and how environmental factors may interact with genetic factors to influence the development of the disorder. Answering these questions could lead to new insights into the mechanisms behind EDS and potential new treatment targets.

Overall, while EDS can be a challenging condition to live with, there is reason to be hopeful for the future. Advances in research and treatment offer the potential for new therapies and better management of symptoms, while ongoing research into the underlying causes of the disorder could lead to new breakthroughs in our understanding of EDS. Additionally, increased awareness of EDS and improved diagnostic tools could lead to earlier diagnosis and more effective treatment. While there is still much work to be done, the future of EDS research and treatment looks promising.

Made in the USA
Middletown, DE
15 October 2023

40811051R00033